Get Pregnant

**Helpful Tips To Getting
Pregnant And Overcoming Infertility**

By: Heather Rose

TABLE OF CONTENTS

Publishers Notes

Copyright © 2014 Speedy Publishing LLC

All rights reserved. In accordance with the U.S. Copyright Act of 1976, the scanning, uploading and electronic sharing of any part of this book without the explicit written consent or permission of the publisher constitutes unlawful piracy and the theft of intellectual property.

If you would like to use material or consent from this book (other than for review purposes), prior written permission must be obtained from the publisher.

You can contact the publishing company at admin@speedypublishing.com. Thank you for not infringing on the author's rights.

Speedy Publishing LLC

40 E. Main St., #1156

Newark, DE 19711

www.speedypublishing.co

Manufactured in the United States of America.

This is a **reprint** book

DEDICATION

This book is dedicated to those who are struggling with infertility and desiring to become a parent.

Introduction

Far too many people struggle to fall pregnant and conceive a child naturally. This generally drives most people to visit a doctor or specialist to find out why they have so much trouble conceiving and giving birth to healthy, happy babies.

In most cases, they're given a diagnosis of infertility.

Unfortunately, there are many different reasons for infertility, so this doesn't always help. It's known that ovarian cysts, PCOS and endometriosis can affect your fertility rate, as can a low sperm count. Some people are affected by other hormonal issues or more complicated problems, such as blocked or obstructed fallopian tubes.

Even with all the advances made by medical science, there still remains a possibility that doctors simply can't find a cause for some peoples' infertility problems. Yet what most people forget is that traditional, natural remedies often have a far greater success rate than expensive, often painful medical treatments.

Despite a higher success rate, many people choose to ignore natural treatments and solutions that really could prepare your body to conceive naturally, even after being told that you're infertile by a medical specialist.

In fact, it's been proven that some fertility treatments prescribed by fertility specialists can increase the risk of contracting ovarian cancer, yet women every day still opt to take expensive medications rather than consider some of the more healthy options of trying a holistic approach.

What's more, many of the medical treatments, surgeries and pharmaceutical drugs for infertility don't actually treat the base cause of the problem. Instead, they treat the symptom and attempt to remove it that way. This can sometimes cause more problems than you started with.

This book will look at some reasons for infertility and how using a natural, holistic approach to reversing your infertility problems can greatly improve your chances of conceiving a child of your own without surgery and without drugs.

Are you ready to change your life and become a happy parent?

Chapter 1 – Infertility In Women

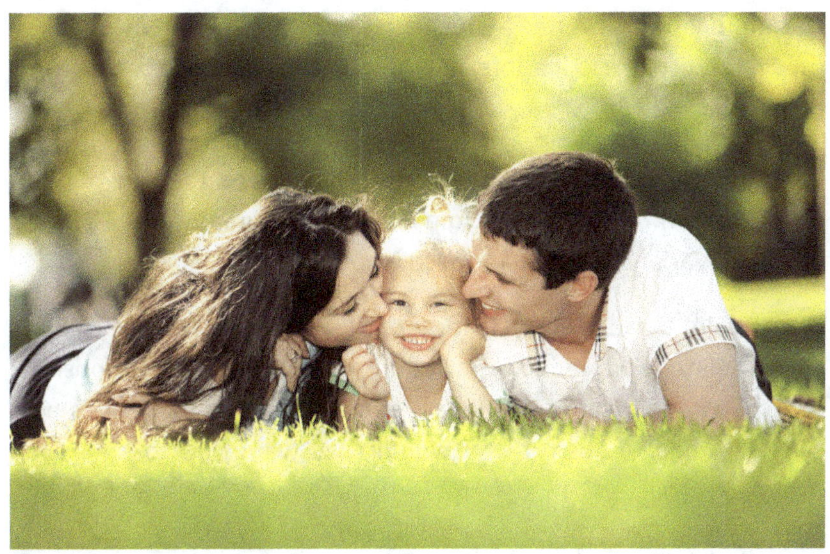

There are so many different reasons for infertility, in both men and women, that it's impossible to use a blanket term to cover everything. Instead, it's important to look at various things that could affect your chances of conceiving and consider what diagnosis suits your own personal situation.

Ovarian Cysts

Ovarian cysts are small fluid-filled sacs that develop in the ovaries. In most cases, they're completely harmless, but they can rupture and cause tremendous pain. If a ruptured cyst is left untreated, it can form sepsis, which is quite toxic and potentially lethal.

Of course, the presence of ovarian cysts can also interfere with normal conception.

Most medical specialists will recommend that any cysts be removed surgically, which can be a painful and expensive procedure. What they don't tell you is that it's possible to reduce ovarian cysts naturally and painlessly.

'Lazy' Ovaries

Some specialists will diagnose 'lazy' ovaries as a cause of infertility. This simply means an egg isn't being released when it should, so they'll tend to prescribe infertility drugs, such as Clomid, to induce ovulation.

Unfortunately, studies in Washington have proved that the number of women who had taken Clomid are three times more likely to develop ovarian cancer than those who don't.

Once again, these specialists forget to let you know there are ways to stimulate and induce ovulation using natural methods. Of course, when you consider that the infertility drug industry is now a billion dollar industry, why would they want you to know you could do it yourself?

PCOS (PolyCystic Ovarian Syndrome)

Polycystic Ovarian Syndrome is the term given when many small cysts are apparent within the ovaries. PCOS is thought to be one of the leading causes of female infertility. In some cases, this can be linked to obesity, acne, increased insulin resistance, lack of ovulation and sometimes an excess of masculinizing hormones.

Of course, this doesn't mean every patient who has acne or who is obese will have PCOS. Similarly, patients who have ovarian cysts may not have PCOS.

Similarly, patients showing an excess of masculinizing hormones may show unwanted facial and body hair growth as well as developing acne, but they also may not have PCOS.

Correct diagnosis can sometimes be difficult, but treatment can be relatively easy with prescription of a dietary supplement known as DCI, which is a naturally occurring human metabolite that helps with insulin metabolism.

Endometriosis

Endometriosis is the medical name given when the uterine lining that would normally shed as part of a regular monthly menstrual cycle grows on the outside of the uterus instead of inside. This is a major cause of infertility in women.

Endometriosis can cause very painful menstrual periods, as well as heavy bleeding and can be responsible for repeated miscarriages.

Infertility Specialists recommend laparoscopic surgery to remove the endometrial lining and any abnormal tissue, however, there are plenty of alternative natural therapies available to remedy this problem.

There are plenty of success stories from patients with endometriosis using traditional Chinese medicine, including traditional herbalism and acupuncture.

Fallopian Tube Blockages

Blocked or damaged fallopian tubes are thought to account for up to 40% of female infertility problems. Blocked tubes will prevent eggs reaching the uterus and prevent sperm from reaching the egg. In most cases, women have no idea their tubes might be blocked, as there are generally no obvious symptoms to look for. Blocked fallopian tubes are generally diagnosed by pelvic ultrasound, although a hysterosalpinogram may also be used, in which a dye is placed into the cervix before x-raying the pelvic region.

There are two types of blocked tubes – partial blockage and Hydrosalpinx.

A partial blockage may be a result of endometrial lining closing off a portion of the tube, which can result in a tubal pregnancy, or ectopic pregnancy. A hydrosalpinx is when the tube is completely blocked and begins to fill with fluid, which makes the tube dilate and swell as it fills. If both tubes are affected, the chances of conceiving are zero.

The predominant causes of blocked tubes are a history of Pelvic Inflammatory Disease, Chlamydia, ruptured appendix, endometriosis or other type of uterine infection.

Infertility specialists will advise that laparoscopic surgery is required to unblock the affected tubes, however this can cause further scarring in some cases. In the case of a hydrosalpinx, a specialist may advise that a hydrosalpingectomy is required, which is complete removal of the dilated fallopian tube. This destroys any chance of falling pregnant naturally in future and the patient becomes dependent on IVF treatments if further children are wanted.

Once again, there are plenty of non-surgical options available to help unblock damaged fallopian tubes. Alternative therapies that include manual physical therapy have also shown positive results.

CHAPTER 2- INFERTILITY IN MEN

Most people are simply unaware that around 35-40% of all infertility problems are because of the male. It's almost instantly assumed that the female must be having some kind of problems.

Yet male infertility is almost as high as female infertility. Some of the common causes of male infertility are widely recognized, such as low sperm count, but there are others that aren't quite so well-known.

Low Sperm Count

Low sperm count or poor sperm mobility can cause infertility. There are many biological and environmental factors that can cause a low sperm count.

Age is a factor in sperm production, with a 60% fertilization rate evident in men younger than 39, but only a 30% fertilization rate for men older than 40.

However, factors such as stress, impotence and premature ejaculation can reduce sperm counts as well. In these cases, it could be wise to work on ways to reduce stress levels and work on the mental and emotion causes behind impotence and premature ejaculation before considering medical treatments.

Substance abuse and smoking are well known to both impair sperm count and reduce mobility drastically. It's also been proven that men who smoke have far lower sex drives, so have sex less frequently.

Men who have poor diets or who have specific deficiencies in vitamin C, selenium, zinc or folate are at far greater risk for low sperm count.

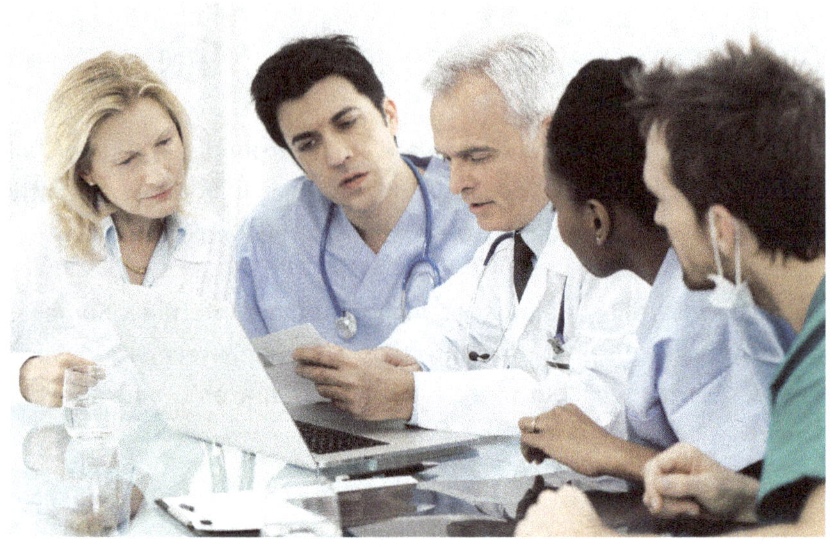

Overheating the testicles can cause temporary low sperm counts and this can be caused by things like saunas, hot tubs, high fever or even wearing underwear that causes the testicles to sit too close to the heat of the body. Combat this by wearing boxer shorts.

Surprisingly, one of the leading causes of impotence and infertility in men is bicycling. This is because pressure from the bike seat can damage sensitive blood vessels and nerves that cause erections and conduct blood flow to the perineum (the area between the scrotum and the anus). This can damage the testicles and scrotum, reducing sperm production.

Infertility specialists will happily prescribe drugs and medication to increase sperm count and boost sperm production. Incidentally, these are similar to those that stimulate ovulation. Side effects of drugs such as clomiphene and hMG can cause blurred vision, weight gain and even liver damage.

Yet there are many, many natural ways to increase sperm count without resorting to drugs or medications.

Male Tube Blockages

Infertility in men can sometimes be caused by tubal blockages in the vas deferens or epididymis (these are the tubes that transport sperm).

The most common cause of male tube blockage is varicose veins within the testicles. However, some sexually transmitted diseases, such as Chlamydia or gonorrhea can also cause blockage problems.

Doctors will recommend surgery to repair the varicoceles, but it should be noted that it can take between 6 and 9 months before a male will be able to impregnate a woman after the surgery.

Once again, there are plenty of natural treatments that can help to rectify these problems, yet far too many people don't even consider them.

Non-Specific Infertility

Of course, there are a percentage of couples who are diagnosed with 'non-specific infertility'. These are the couples where nothing specific can be located to explain why conception isn't happening.

Despite months of trying to conceive and subsequent months of tests, trials and specialist's appointments, many couples still don't have a logical explanation for why they can't fall pregnant.

When OB-GYNs and infertility specialists run a battery of tests, they're medically based. They look for hormonal imbalances. They look for the obvious signs of blocked tubes, cysts, sperm quality and quantity and other usual signs that something might be wrong that they can fix with medications or surgery.

Unfortunately, when they can't find anything logical, it's categorized as 'non-specific infertility' and they tend to resort to putting the couple onto fertility drugs like Clomid to see if that will help.

What they forget is the enormous range of other factors that can affect fertility that have nothing to do with the obvious symptoms the majority of people tend to display.

Our bodies are designed to send out warning signals when something is wrong. These signals are usually displayed as pain or symptoms or other issues that need to be addressed in order to fix the cause.

Unfortunately, the multi-billion dollar pharmaceutical industry would much rather treat the symptoms rather than work on ways to fix the cause of the problem in the first place.

By taking pain relief medication, you're actually masking the real warning sign your body is trying to give you. By taking infertility drugs, you're denying that your body is sending out a message that something is wrong with your reproductive system that needs to be addressed first, before you conceive your child.

This can sometimes lead to making the original problem even worse in the long run.

Chapter 3- Understanding The Human Body

The human body is an amazingly complex thing. Biologically, we're designed to run efficiently by ingesting nutritious foods that give us the energy to exert ourselves physically, but also to fuel the neurons that fire within our brains.

Our brains are hundreds of times more complex than the most advanced computers on the planet. A brain is capable of keeping your body running on unconscious actions, such as breathing, or keeping your heart pumping, but it's also capable of releasing various hormones that help us to cope with everything we face during the day.

Your own body will release certain hormones to let you know its tired, different hormones when it's time to wake up, more hormones when you're feeling happy and different ones again when you're stressed or upset.

That's not even counting the myriad of hormones, enzymes and other goodies your brain releases to tell your body it's the optimum time to release an egg from one of your ovaries at the right time for your body to conceive.

So what happens when those hormones aren't released at the right time or in the right amounts?

In most cases, people tend to visit their doctor and come home with a prescription for drugs to help regulate those hormones. What they don't know is those chemical cocktails can sometimes cause other issues with the smooth functioning of your body, even while they might be addressing the initial problem you sought to fix.

Well-Oiled Machine

Think for a moment about how your body might be a little like a car. If you put the wrong type of gasoline into your car's tank, it's not likely to run very well. If you put cooking oil instead of motor oil into the engine, it's very likely to break down completely.

Now think about what you put into your own tank each and every day to keep your motor running.

You might think you're eating enough food to sustain you on a daily basis, but really think about what nutritional value you're adding into those meals.

Once again, to use the car analogy, if you were to fill your car's gas tank with water, it would be full – but it won't be full of what it needs to run properly.

The same is true with your body.

In order to really function properly and really respond to any kind of infertility treatments, you need to overhaul your current nutritional plan.

Look at some ways you can cut out the processed foods and replace it with healthier options. Are there any ways you could increase the nutrients you consume by replacing a few simple things?

Of course, it's also worth looking at what else you're putting into your body's tank. Things like caffeine, nicotine, alcohol and drugs can also reduce your chances of conceiving naturally, as they affect the normal functions of your body.

There are plenty of ways to add more nutritional value to your diet each day, but it's still important to realize why you're doing it.

Fighting the Blues

Did you know that researchers have found a link between high stress levels in women and infertility? When women suffer from stress, they release testosterone into their systems.

This can make them seem more aggressive, more upset, more moody and definitely less able to cope with the pressures of life without reaching breaking point.

To counteract these stress hormones, women need to release oxytocin, which reduces stress levels and brings about a sense of being in a loving, nurturing life.

Learning to combat stress effectively can play an important role in reversing infertility, as too much testosterone in your system can reduce the chances of you releasing the right pregnancy hormones you need to fall pregnant.

Reducing and Eliminating Toxins

Think about the enormous number of chemicals, toxins and other poisons we're exposed to each and every day of our lives. Even the products we use to clean the environments in which we live are nothing more than harsh, harmful chemicals.

If you knew you were cleaning your shower or toilet with chemicals that could be affecting your fertility rate, would you change brands? Will another brand actually have the same types of chemicals in it?

What about the shampoo and conditioner you use? They might make your hair feel and smell lovely, but do you know what the chemicals inside those products are made from – or what else they're used for?

Have you ever wondered why we're taught to spit out toothpaste after we've brushed our teeth instead of just swallowing the minty-tasting foam?

There are so many simple, routine things we do each and every day that could potentially be increasing the level of toxins in your body.

Of course, there are some other types of toxins that aren't so noticeable. Things like mercury levels in some types of fish can also affect your body's optimal function.

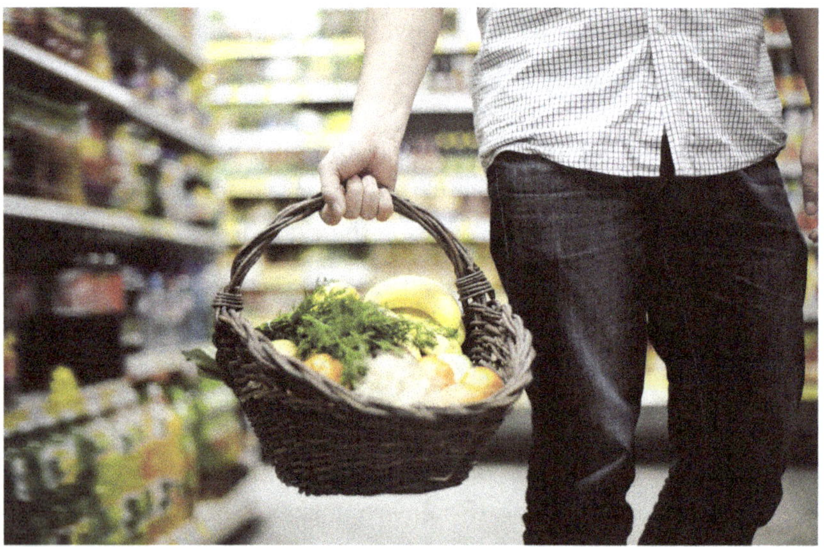

Foods to Avoid When Trying to Conceive

If you're already having trouble conceiving, you should consider cutting down on certain foods, or eliminating them from your diet altogether.

It's a well-known fact that caffeine intake can reduce your fertility rate by up to 50%. While you might think this means cutting out that coffee each morning, it's important to realize how many other foods and beverages contain hidden amounts of caffeine that could be affecting your ovulation rate and your hormonal balances.

Things like chocolate and soda also contain caffeine. There are also some pain relievers that contain amounts of caffeine, such as Anacin and Excedrin. It's important to read labels if you're unsure of anything just to rule out those hidden sources of caffeine.

Alcohol is also detrimental to your fertility rate. Eliminate it from your diet by as much as four months before conceiving. The same is true for smoking.

Optimizing Your Health

When you improve your diet, your body is far more able to generate the right levels and types of hormones you need to feel good, be healthy and respond very well to infertility treatments.

You may also find that a relaxed 30 minute walk each day could increase your health even further. You'll be outside, which increases your Vitamin D intake and you'll be exercising moderately, which boosts your endorphin levels.

You may also find you begin to lose weight and have far more energy throughout the day.

There are plenty of health benefits to be had by eating the right kinds of foods with the correct levels of nutrition, vitamins and minerals, but the real importance is your own biological awareness.

You see, your brain may be choosing not to release the right hormones into your system in order for you to get pregnant naturally until it feels as though the right environment has been created to nurture an embryo to term.

What's more, it's been shown in several medical studies that improving your diet and lifestyle can actually reduce ovarian cysts and reduce menstrual cramps.

Of course, improving your diet and hormonal levels are only one aspect of beating infertility. There are plenty of other considerations to think about, too.

Foods to Add to Your Diet When Trying to Conceive

It's been well-documented that foods that are low in fat and high in fiber will help to increase your body's overall health. Add simple things into your diet that include fruits, legumes, vegetables and nuts, as well as sensible choices for lean meat or chicken.

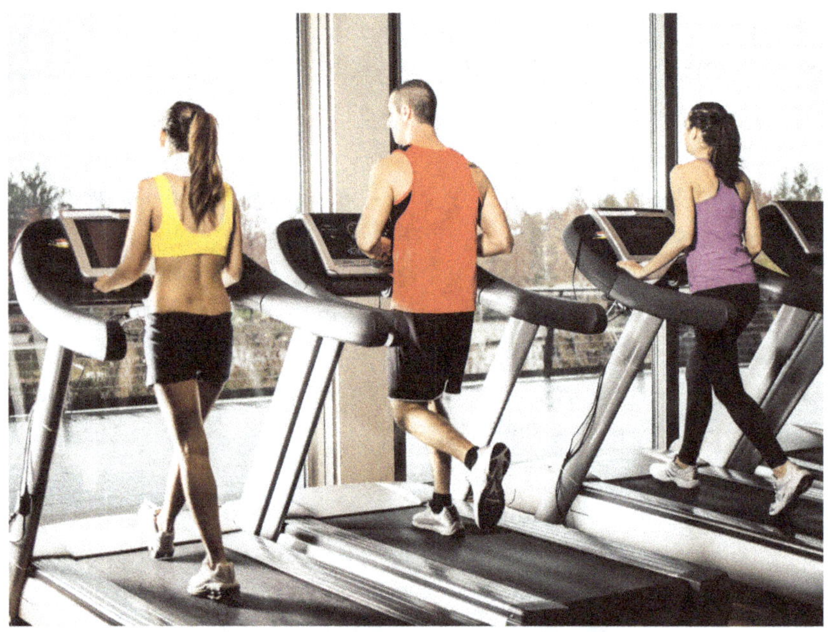

Finding foods that contain natural sources of folic acid and Vitamin B will also help to boost your natural immune system and help you to create a viable environment for conception to take place. Folic acid also helps to prevent birth defects, like spina bifida, and can also help reduce the incidence of miscarriage.

Some good natural sources of folic acid and vitamin B are green leafy vegetables, avocado, asparagus, papaya, broccoli, eggs, oranges, nuts, beans and wheat breads.

Oysters are also high on the list of foods to add to improve fertility, as they have a high zinc factor. It's well documented that males and females with zinc deficiencies may experience reduced fertility levels, so oysters can help.

Of course, just adding one or two types of foods to your diet might improve your chances of conceiving a little, but they won't cure infertility. A well-balanced diet, coupled with moderate exercise will help improve your overall health and hormonal levels.

CHAPTER 4- TALKING ABOUT SEX

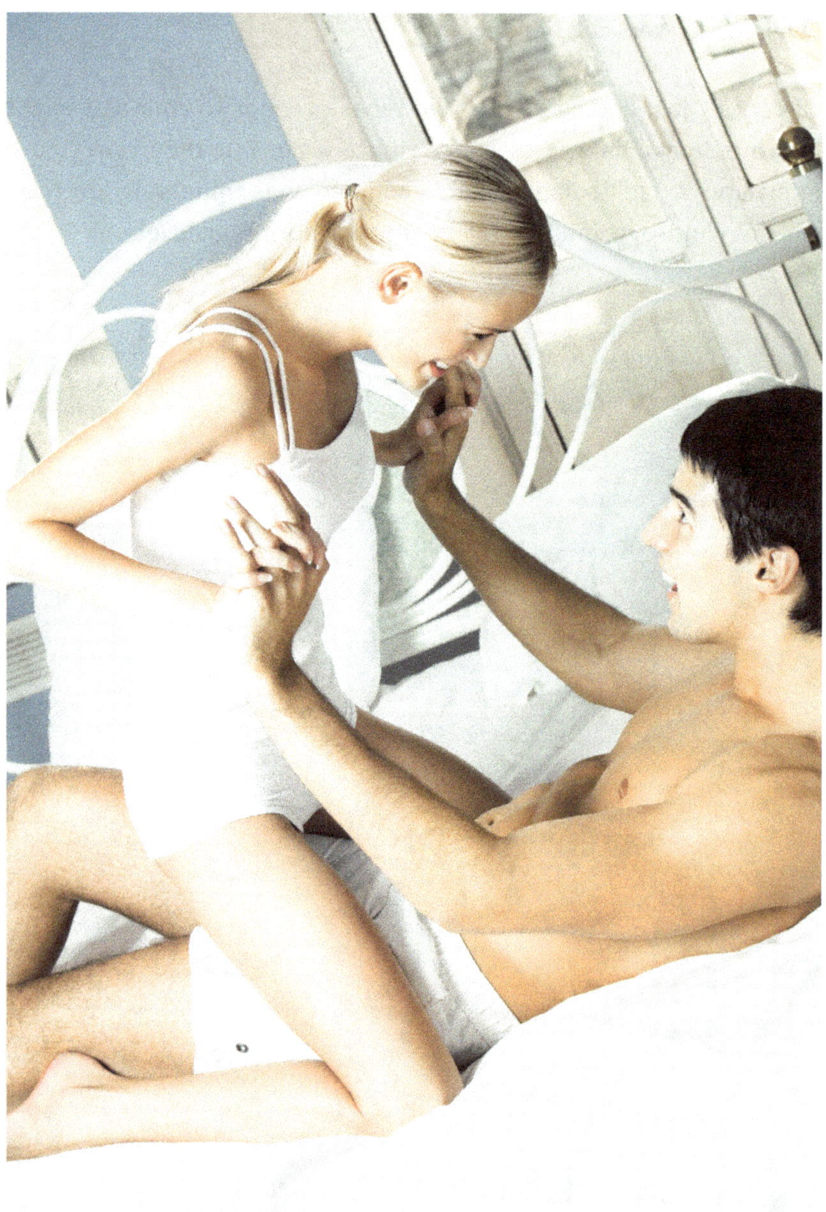

There is a lot of misinformation around about when you should have sex in order to improve your chances of conceiving. In schools, teenagers are taught that they could have sex at any time during their cycle and fall pregnant, but this is not accurate.

The best time to have sex in order to conceive is ideally 2-3 days before you ovulate. This is your most fertile time and you have the highest chances of conceiving before you actually release an egg.

Of course, this leads to the problem of knowing exactly when you're going to ovulate in the first place.

Ideally, a monthly menstrual cycle should last 28 days, with day one being the first day of your period. Some doctors state that ovulation is usually on day 14 of a menstrual cycle, so many women decide to plan to have sex on day 14, hoping to increase their chances of getting pregnant.

The problem with this approach is that not every woman has an exact 28 day cycle. Similarly, not every woman will ovulate on exactly day 14. You might ovulate on day 10 or on day 17.

There are ways to predict ovulation using basal body temperature kits or ovulation predictor kits, both of which are available at most pharmacies.

However, the single most reliable predictor of when you're at your most fertile point of the month is on the day you notice the most fertile cervical mucus discharge.

Cervical mucus is the discharge that is sticky, clear and a little like raw egg white. Having sex when you notice the cervical mucus is important, simply because this discharge is what aids sperm in surviving and swimming to the egg more effectively.

Timing When to Have Sex

Unfortunately, when many women decide to put off having sex until they notice their cervical mucus discharge, they tend to abstain completely until it's the "right time". They also tend to avoid sex at other times during the cycle.

This can mean sex becomes a chore or a routine. It becomes less about love and connection, which can increase strain on a relationship and increase stress levels for both of you.

Of course, you may also find that, even though the woman might be at her peak fertility time, you could be reducing the male's sperm quality without even knowing it.

You see, if you wait to have sex for a week or two before you notice the signs of ovulation, you risk your partner's sperm quality being at less than peak quality.

This is because a male's sperm quality and quantity will peak after only one or two days of abstinence. If you've made him wait for 10, the quality and quantity may not be ideal for optimum fertility rates.

Ideally, if you're planning to conceive, having sex twice a week, regardless of the fertility signs can actually strengthen the connection between you, as well as increase fertility for each of you at the same time.

Stop timing when to have sex and work on having a little fun together instead.

Good Sex = Better Chances of Conception

As mentioned in the previous section, many women become so preoccupied in trying to figure out the right time of the month to have sex that they forget about having fun and enjoying it.

When you have sex based on a calendar or a time table, it can lose a lot of the 'fun' factor. This can build resentment and cause stress, which can become a factor in keeping you infertile.

Researchers have shown that women who orgasm during sex can increase their chances of falling pregnant. This is because the spasmodic contractions of the uterus can actually help pull the sperm further into the uterus rather than remaining in the vagina where it can leak out far more easily.

Sex Positions

Yes, there are some sexual positions that are naturally going to help your chances of conception better than others. Of course, it's still possible to get pregnant with any position at all. However, some positions may help increase your chances.

Keep in mind that if a woman enjoys sex on top, this could reduce the chances of as much sperm getting to where it needs to go. Gravity plays a part here, so if you're on top, the sperm is going to leak out more easily.

For the more adventurous types, you might be a little disappointed to hear that missionary position is still the leading favorite position for optimal conception.

Ideally, place a pillow under your hips to tilt your pelvis up, but be sure the pillow isn't too large, as you don't want the sperm pooling behind your cervix. This will also help keep the sperm in longer and give the sperm more time to easily swim up through the cervix where it needs to go to reach the egg. Don't get up immediately after sex to wash or wipe, either. Allow the sperm to stay in for as long as possible.

However, if you have a tipped uterus, you may find that the "doggy position" might be more beneficial for you. Go ahead and get onto your hands and knees, and encourage your partner to enter from behind. He'll have fun and you'll be increasing your chances of getting that sperm where it needs to go.

There's still a lot of fun to be had experimenting with variations on the missionary position without reducing your conception odds. See what you and your partner can come up with to work on ways to add spice to the missionary position to increase the fun factor, while still remaining in the right position for the most possible sperm to reach your uterus.

CHAPTER 5- BOY OR GIRL?

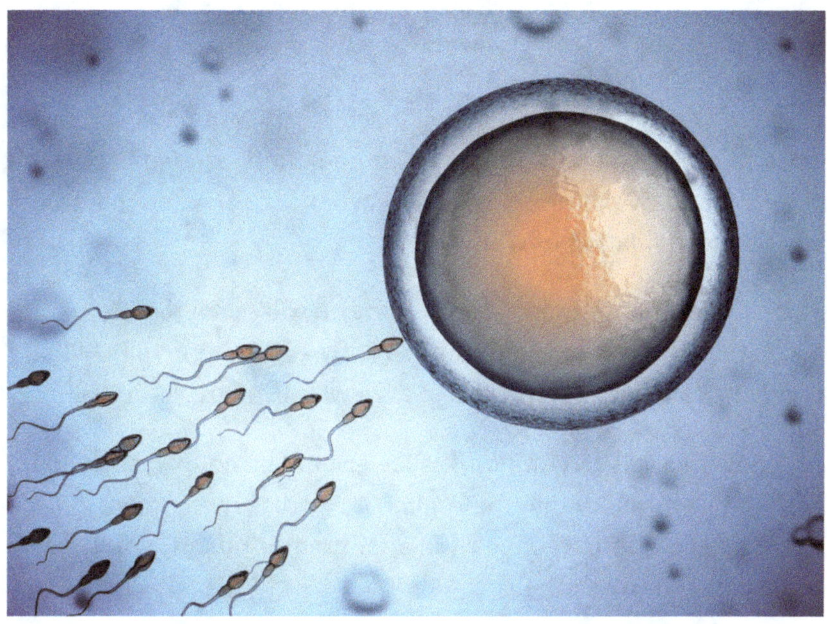

There is a preconception that having sex at a certain time or eating certain foods or having sex in a particular position might increase your chances of conceiving a boy or a girl.

While there are some suggestions that you can increase your chances of conceiving a baby of a particular sex during certain times of your ovulation period, these are not foolproof.

When you consider that a male will ejaculate millions of sperm upon orgasm, trying to aim at one specific type of these is going to be a hit and miss operation.

Basically, men produce two types of sperm: an X and a Y. The slower, larger X sperm will become female, while the faster, smaller Y sperm will be male.

This is where timing when you have sex becomes important.

Keep in mind there is no guaranteed way to determine the sex of your baby, but you can work on ways to favor your odds for or against one or the other.

Trying for a Girl

If you're trying for a girl, you will need to try and have sex seven days before ovulation and then every day until around 3 or more days prior to ovulation. Then try to avoid sex for a few days until you're sure ovulation is over.

This is because the smaller, faster Y sperm will reach the uterus and die before the egg is even released. However, there will still be a number of slower, larger X sperm alive when you ovulate.

Another theory is to work on shallower penetration. This has to do with the pH levels within the vagina. An acidic environment will kill the weaker Y sperm first, leaving a far greater quantity of X sperm remaining to fertilize the egg.

Besides, with deeper penetration, the sperm is deposited much closer to the egg, which can mean the faster Y sperm may reach their destination before the X sperm can.

You may also decrease the acidity levels within the vagina if you reach orgasm during sex. If you're trying for a girl, it may be best not to reach orgasm, as your body will release a substance that could make the vagina more alkaline instead of acidic.

Trying for a Boy

When trying for a boy, it may become important to try and not have sex until you reach around 2-3 days before ovulation. Then have sex every day until after ovulation has occurred.

Sex should involve deep penetration to deposit the sperm as close as possible to the cervix, and work towards having an orgasm during sex to pull even more sperm into the womb for better success.

It's also been noted that, while women should not drink any caffeine while drinking to conceive, one strong cup of coffee prior to sex for the MAN could actually increase the motility of the Y sperm, increasing your chances of having a boy.

CONCLUSION

There is no single magic pill or solution that can cure your infertility, but there are plenty of ways to improve your health, reduce cysts and blocked tubes, and remedy your hormonal imbalances that will greatly improve your chances of conceiving naturally.

Look into natural methods to address the specific reasons behind your own infertility and you'll find there shouldn't be a need for painful surgery or expensive medications with dangerous side-effects.

It is possible to reduce ovarian cysts on your own. You really can unblock your own blocked fallopian tubes and you really can amend any hormonal problems you might have faced simply by understanding how to balance natural treatments with a balanced diet and the right type of exercise.

You should also find that when you begin working on simple dietary changes, along with a little extra exercise, you will feel more energetic and look younger. You'll feel happier and less depressed. You'll experience less mood swings.

You may also find that you don't suffer from PMS or bloating or cramps nearly as much. And if you had problems with hormonal imbalances, you should find that unwanted facial hair goes away. You'll reduce acne breakouts and your skin and hair will develop a new vitality.

On top of all this, you'll be creating a healthy, conducive body that will become a prime environment to conceive your own child.

Good luck and happy parenting.

ABOUT THE AUTHOR

Heather Rose is an expert for both physical and mental health with years of practice to back it up. From her own experience of working with those who are experiencing the parenting problems of various degrees, she now shares her knowledge of dealing to a large audience.

She writes on various strategies on managing individuals with such problems and how to help their lives more enjoyable and much less stressful and frustrating. It also makes life easier for the family and the people around them cope with their symptoms.